The Transformative Power of Self-Care

By

Tiffany Alston and LaShonda Jack

Editor: Jeanette Lenoir

Cover Concept: Tiffany Alston and
LaShonda Jack

Cover Design: Brittany J. Jackson

Published by G Publishing, LLC

ISBN: 979-8-9876534-0-1

Library of Congress Control Number:
2023901795

Printed in the United States of America

CONTENTS

DEDICATIONS

I would like to dedicate this book to my children, Timothy, Timora & Timple. Your constant love and support activate the Superhero in me. Also, this book would not be possible without the greatest friendship any woman could have. My best friend Tiffany Alston. Thank you for motivating me, keeping me on task and always seeing the greatest parts of who I am. Your friendship and business partnership is second to none.

I dedicate this book to those who are longing for sincere change, never to remain the same. As you read through the pages, exploring with curiosity, I wish for you to feel inspired, to be transformed with a renewed sense of purpose. While also having the freedom, knowledge and understanding that self-care begins with you. Self-Care is not selfish; it's for everyone. You are the true MVP (Most Valuable Person) of your life.

LaShonda Jack

I am grateful that God has allowed me to write this book. I dedicate this book to my husband Donald Alston, and our three sons Christopher, Christian & Cameron Alston. Family is one of life's greatest blessings, love you all. I also would like to dedicate this book to you, the reader. I wish you peace and blessings as you begin your new self-care journey or continue in it. I want to encourage you to take care of your mind, body and soul; by embracing life to the fullest throughout your transformation.

Last but not least, I dedicate this book to my best friend and business partner Shonda Jack. Thank you for showing me what sisterhood truly means. I'm grateful to have crossed paths with you three years ago and developed this wonderful friendship. In life we were able to write this book together. God bless all of you!

Tiffany Alston

INTRODUCTION

The self-care movement was founded by none other than Socrates the legendary Greek philosopher from the 5th century. He became known as one to question power, he taught those seeking power to first work on themselves. The philosophical thought at that time was about caring for your soul and knowing thyself first. To train your mind and build your body for alignment before one can be capable of comprehending truth.

Socrates believed it was his God given purpose to teach people how to take care of themselves and feed their souls. Socrates presented a question Are you not ashamed for devoting all your care to increasing wealth, reputation and honor while not caring for or even considering your reason, truth and constant improvement of self? However, this ideology cost him his life. After his death Plato another Greek philosopher, also a student of Socrates suggested that self-care led to enlightenment as well as political success. During that time period early Christians believed that self-care was about celibacy and abandoning all possessions in order to get to a higher self- actualization. When that era ended the dark ages came into higher dimensions of philosophical thought centered around self-care.

It wasn't until the 1950's that self-care re-emerged throughout the medical community and was seen as an alternative path to health and wellness for those in the medical community; to encourage patients to treat themselves. This became a new medical practice for patients to proactively cultivate a sense of self-worth through care and preservation. Self-Care began to make its way throughout academic circles as a way for academia to better understand post-traumatic stress in various people groups. In the 1960's community civil rights leaders of the Black Panther Party Huey P. Newton & Bobby Seale, viewed self-care as means to change the narrative for the BIPOC community

(Black, Indigenous, People of Color) it served. They saw self-care as a resource of freedom and liberation while fighting against social injustice within marginalized communities. This started a self-care revolution because they saw self-care as a means for survival within their community. The lack of access to basic health, and social services caused by systematic barriers during that time became fuel for the movement. Self-Care practice evolved within the community to counter burn-out and compassion fatigue. Programs were developed to educate people on eating healthier, to care for their physical bodies though exercises such as yoga. Mindfulness & meditations was highly encouraged by instructors Angela Davis & Erica Huggins. Together wellness programs were developed to help preserve mental health in the communities as well to aid them in navigating social, political and equitable systems; also known as radical self-care. To bring one's entire self into the movement; to embody self-care in the work as an activist by acknowledging and moving beyond trauma, with a holistic approach was the mission.

1980s French philosopher Michale Vocoall said, "One should take heed to self by applying their mind to self as well as being aware of your qualities." In the same decade, writer and poet Audra Lorde said, "Caring for myself is not self- "indulgent, it's self-preservation, bringing awareness to the intersectionality of self-care and civil rights."

Her writings highlighted self-preservation as foundational for building a community; spanning boundaries. Self-Care is about doing the work by examining and improving yourself in order to better serve the world in which you live. We believe self-care is a historical shift; taking place in our society right now at this very moment. It's time to look after our mental health. Putting your needs first, will have a positive effect on everything in your life including your relationships and tolerance. Self-Care has restorative powers; it refills your cup in order to properly pour into others around you. It facilitates your contributions to society in such a way that aligns with your core values; for you to make a difference.

Self-Care is here to help you in making the right choices for the long-term and short term of things. Your self-care practice will inspire others around you. They will become fans because of your results and your way of reducing the risks of self-harm. Ultimately you will be the inspiration of a new way of being and they will want to be the same.

CHAPTER 1
Self-Care 101

Self-Care is the practice of taking care of yourself by doing the things that will feed your soul, nurture your body and uplift your spirit. Implementing these behaviors can promote a healthy lifestyle along with wellness and self-management. Having a daily self- care routine has been proven to reduce stress, eliminate anxiety, depression, minimal frustration, anger, improve energy and increase happiness. Regarding self-care,

this is simply about filling your own cup;
to the levels of which you can pour out to
others. You can't give out of an empty
cup!

Many benefits come with having a
self-care practice because self-care is for
everyone. Relationships are greatly
improved when you take care of
yourself. For example, a person becomes
more authentic, empathetic, well
balanced, and has meaningful
connections.

Satisfaction is another benefit to taking care of yourself. Moments in life are enjoyable due to having those healthy relationships. What does a healthy relationship look like for you? They should include,

- Mutual respect

- Compromise

- Honesty

- Good communication

- Understanding

- Trust

- Acceptance

- Boundaries

Self-esteem is boosted, leaving you feeling more self-confident, nurturing mental health. When self-esteem is high, you no longer dwell on the past or negative experiences. You're able to express your needs while maintaining a positive outlook on life. You appreciate your strengths and weaknesses for what they are, as well as knowing when to say no. Physically your body responds to all things positively. Physical wellness involves exercise, making healthy food and drink choices. They will make you feel amazing giving you the balance of nutrition and energy needed just for you. Also, it's important to ensure that you develop a healthy night cap routine, for a time of relaxation and a great night's sleep.

On this journey as you begin to explore self-care, you'll notice changes in your emotions. As you lean in you will find out more about who you are. Also new skill sets will emerge such as kindness, compassion, the ability to have difficult conversations, be more resilient, and overcome challenges that arise in our daily lives. To get started with this practice, you'll need to develop a healthy self-care routine.

For starters, set your intention for self-care practice. This is known as your "Why". Next carve out some time each day for you. This could be anywhere from 20-30 minutes up to 1 hour. No worries, the intention is to start. Focus on consistency while considering your mind, body, & spirit. Find an accountability partner. This could be someone who will support you and not judge you. Celebrate your micro and macro successes. Incorporate journaling this will help you to connect with those inner thoughts and feelings where you feel safe to clear the mind. Remember, self- care looks different for everyone. It depends on your lifestyle, faith background, gender, age and your environment.

CHAPTER 2
Taking Care of Your Body

Many years ago, there was a commercial on T.V. that showed people drinking milk. During that segment the commercial would always end with the tagline "Milk does a body good." Studies have shown that it's sleep; that does a body good. Getting sleep increases your productivity, focus, energy, and concentration. The quality of sleep impacts how your immune system functions. As you sleep, the immune system releases a protein called cytokine. Some cytokines need to increase when there is infection, inflammation, and stress present.

The lack of sleep also inhibits the recovery time from illnesses   such as unknown viruses and common colds. Sleep deprivation causes a reduction in infection-fighting antibodies cells. Long-term sleep reduction increases the risk of diabetes, obesity, heart disease or blood vessel disease. It's been proven that as you get the proper rest it decreases the chance of experiencing insomnia, mood disorders, anxiety, depression and panic attacks. Approximately 8 hours of sleep per night is suggested for adults.

Drinking water and eating healthy allows the body to function efficiently. When you're properly hydrated, your skin and hair look healthier. Drinking water can prevent dehydration, which causes unclear thinking, constipation, and kidney stones. Water also helps your body flush out toxins. Drinking water doesn't have to be boring. It can be a fun hydration experience when you add fruits, vegetables and herbs to it. We call it Self- Care H2O!

Good nutrition is self-care because your relationship with healthy food can create a sense of balance in your life. Food is fuel for the body. Yet it depends on how balanced your nutritional intake and portion sizes are. Adding spices while cooking your food is also self-care. While cooking your food, you reduce levels of chemicals, sodium, cholesterol, calories, fiber, water content, and other fats while increasing nutrients. Eating when you feel hungry keeps your emotions intact and blood sugar stable.

Starting with your plate and the foods that you eat, is a great way to weave self-care into your daily routine. One way to practice self -care with food is mindful eating. With mindful eating you are bringing your full attention to your food. Starting with a small portion of the food, you will offer up appreciation for it; pausing for 1 minute or 2 minutes to think about everything

and everyone it took to bring the meal to
your table. Next as you're cooking, bring
all your senses to the meal, noticing all
the colors, textures, the aroma, and
different sounds that the food is making
as you cook. Then take a small bite, as
you chew your food try identifying all
the ingredients and spices used in the
meal. Next, place your utensils down on
the table next to the plate between
bites. Chew your food well until you can
taste the full essence of the delicious
meal. Eat slowly, before bringing your

full attention back to your plate. It is suggested to practice mindful eating for at least 5 minutes before engaging with others at the table.

Engaging in exercise gives everyone a boost. It can be especially helpful in alleviating symptoms. Physical activity allows us to take care of our bodies and minds. Exercise has many benefits including but not limited to,

- Helping to manage weight

- Strengthen muscles and bones

- Reduce the risks of chronic disease

- Manage blood sugar

- Increase longevity

- Improve Sleep

- Mood improvement

- And so much more

There are many forms of exercise such as walking, aerobics, yoga, dancing, swimming, cycling, weightlifting, hiking, tai chi, running, and pilates.

Getting a massage can help you experience ultimate self-care. A massage allows you time to focus on your needs, your thoughts, your feelings and yourself. Massage therapy helps to rebalance hormones and release muscle tension. If you're experiencing a high level of stress, it's likely that your muscles are permanently tensed. Research has shown that massage therapy can reduce cortisol which is a major stress hormone by 31%.

CHAPTER 3
Taking Care of Your Mind

Mindful breathing is an excellent form of self-care. Breathing is the only way that our bodies receive the oxygen that it needs. All our organs depend on the breath. Breathing brings oxygen to the brain. Therefore, when we practice mindful breathing, this sharpens our ability to concentrate. Paying attention to your breath and learning how to alter it, is one way to reduce everyday stress levels, calming the mind and aiding in digestion. When we intentionally breathe deeply, many internal reactions happen such as aids in mental focus, stress reduction, increased joy, and inner enthusiasm.

Let's try it out. Find a comfortable place to sit or lie down, with your feet slightly apart on the ground, place both hands on your lap. Gently inhale slowly through your nose, exhale through your mouth. Focusing on your breath. As you breathe in, imagine warm air flowing through your entire body. Holding the breath for 4 seconds, slowly exhale through your mouth, as if you are blowing out a candle. Repeat until you feel completely relaxed.

To take care of your mind it's important to notice how stress can rewire your brain, by leaving you more vulnerable to experience mental health issues. When we experience emotionally taxing or high stressed situations, the amygdala takes over. The amygdala is the part of your brain that governs your survival instincts. After it's been hijacked, we then experience low energy and are unable to perform necessary tasks.

Emotional resilience is how you cope and adapt to negative or stressful situations. When you experience low levels of emotional resilience, you tend to take things to heart and find it difficult to move on to the next task. High levels of emotional resilience means that you deal with things differently. To boost your emotional resilience, you need to identify the triggers and focus on positive ways to change the response. This allows you to keep those things in perspective without the feeling of anxiousness.

Meditation techniques can help decouple a better sense of inner peace leaving you feeling more confident. Learning to make peace within is the first step in understanding what it means to make peace with all things.

Fear is one of the most paralyzing emotions in our lives. It shows up in various self-conscious forms, i.e., mistrust, doubt. We learn to accept fear with compassion to be explored, be curious enough to understand it and let it go. Letting go is the art of contentment and happiness.

In our lives we face many painful situations where we continue to hold these painful experiences that poisons our capacity to care, whereby we carry them throughout our entire life. Because our hearts have been wounded, we can find ourselves obsessing over and over these experiences that have long passed. This can cause you to live life with regret and bitterness living inside an internal prison. Forgiveness is the key to escape from this internal prison so our hearts can be released from pain. It allows you to live a life in which you no longer carry the burdens from the past. If our hearts and minds are burdened, overfilled or contracted, forging a connection with the natural world is a way of finding greater simplicity and ease.

Human beings have extremely powerful and complex minds. Yet they also have an expansive and complicated sense of self. Because of this their potential to take a lot of things personally, that aren't personal at all.

Humanity has developed an elaborate sense of identity that can make possessions, relationships, conditions and attributes seem as vital to them as their physical survival. For example, someone may be willing to compromise their health and safety in order to maintain a particular physical appearance to compete for a job that gives them status and power.

As complex individuals we are usually engaged in self-referential active thinking. This means that when we are supposedly doing nothing, the brain is highly active. It takes advantage of any down time by analyzing, planning and evaluating all of the stuff in your mind, so you can be better prepared for it. Researchers call this type of thinking stimulus-independent thought.

Connecting with nature is a powerful resource for the wellbeing of self. Surrounding yourself in nature is a remedy for the mind, body and soul. To remain healthy, one must follow the rules of nature.

If done properly the more harmonious you are with it, there's a greater chance of enjoying good health and longevity. When you meditate, your consciousness is opened. A cleansing of the mind will help you to better understand everything that surrounds you. During the practice of meditation, this connection supplies you with pure energy. Meditation opens a new sense of sensitivity and a purer love. Let's try it out.

Find a posture in which your body can be relaxed and upright, shoulders are back with your spine aligned. Take a moment to pause and settle within that posture until you feel a deep sense of ease. Place your feet on the floor, gently close your eyes or look down with a soft gaze. Bringing attention to your breath as your anchor. With each breath notice as you inhale or exhale the rise and fall of your abdomen. Again, gently resting your attention on the breath as your anchor. Next, notice where your attention goes in your mind, whether it's planning things to do, memories, judgment, or daydreaming. Pause, see what's showing up for you in your world of thought, then return your attention to your breathing. For a beginner, this meditation practice should be around 5 minutes or until you feel calm and relaxed with a clear mind.

Self-Love Meditation

Settle into a quiet place, Breath slowly, soften your gaze connecting with your higher self.

Repeat (2x)

May I be safe & protected

May I be happy

May I be healthy & strong

May I be free of physical pain & suffering

May I live in the world peacefully & joyfully with ease

May I be a lover of all things pure

May I care for myself in this ever-changing world gracefully

*May I be resilient when faced
  with challenges*

*May I rest & sleep with natural
  & deeper ease*

*May I be free from mental suffering &
distress*

May I be free from judgment

May I continue to love myself well

CHAPTER 4
8 Elements of Self-Care

Self-Care looks different from person to person. Each element can deliver different benefits when applied.

You may find that some of these elements are more or less nourishing, however always practice what feels good and right for you in that moment. Here's a comprise list of 8 elements for you to activate your self-care wellness routine.

Physical self-care is about movement of the body, health, sleep, and how well you are caring for your physical needs.

Physical Self-Care

- Sleep or rest

- Healthy food

- Exercise

- Attending medical appointments

- Buying new clothing

- Fresh air

- Personal hygiene

- Drink water

Psychological self-care allows you to pay attention to the things that are in your control. As well as your sphere of influence and affluence. This helps to cultivate self- awareness, learning something new and personal growth.

Psychological Self-Care

- Practicing mindfulness

- Listen to a podcast

- Digital detox

- Reading a book

- Say no

- Journal

- Learn a new skill

- Play brain games

Emotional self-care is being able to identify with what you are feeling. When you identify with those feelings, this enables you to honor your true self and emotions.

Emotional Self-Care

- Practicing self-compassion

- Make time to reflect on feelings.

- Talking to a therapist or life coach

- Consciously choose how to respond

- Journaling

- Practice gratitude

- Speak affirmations.

- Ask for help

Social self-care is essential for us. Between work life and home life we rarely find time to really connect with family and friends. Although we connect through technology, it's not the same as having human connections with face-to face interactions.

Social Self-Care

- Going on a date

- Cuddle

- Engage in a community activity

- Spend time with family & friends

- Meet someone new

- Join a social club

- Disconnect from social media

- Schedule social time

Environmental self-care allows you to make small choices every day that will have a huge impact on the world. The environment you're currently in should motivate you, rather than overwhelm, or stress you out.

With the right environment, you will truly thrive.

Environmental Self-Care

- Organize your space

- Designate a work-space

- Add personal touches

- Work in a different environment

- Create a safe space

- Add color

- Rearrange your furniture

- Open windows for fresh air

Professional self-care is having a healthy work life balance. As a professional, you're always expected to multi- task, be productive, while on autopilot. However, this has the potential to lead you towards burnout, overwhelm and chronic stress. Practicing self-care leads to a healthy work life balance.

Professional Self-Care

- Keep work time & personal time separate

- Prioritize your workload

- Take as many breaks as possible when needed

- Use vacation days or sick days

- Form supportive relationships

- Seek new opportunities for growth

- Practice a 3-breath exercise

- Practice mindful eating at lunchtime

Spiritual self-care reassures your belief in a greater sense of purpose and being. Allowing one to make a God connection to ensure that one's faith is strengthened. Spiritual self-care quiets the mind and lessens the turbulence within. It will allow you to get answers to unanswered questions.

<u>**Spiritual Self-Care**</u>

- Pray

- Meditate

- Spend time in nature

- Practice yoga

- Practice forgiveness

- Read an inspirational book

- Serve others in the community

- Listen to inspirational music

Financial self-care supports a healthy money mindset. This is beneficial by helping you to create a better financial future. When working towards your financial goals, you can save, invest, and live debt free.

Financial Self-Care

- Reflect on your relationship with money

- Check accounts regularly

- Create a budget & prioritize debt

- Make investments

- Check credit report

- Enroll in a financial course

- Save

- Invest in others

CHAPTER 5
Trauma, Triggers, Regrets & Letting Go

Developing good self-care habits can be a deep empowering experience for trauma survivors. Trauma is a global issue. Trauma is more than just psychological interdisciplinary, bio-psychosocial phenomenon: It is a public health epidemic. To understand trauma, we must seek to examine its devastating effects. Traumatic experiences vary at the family, community, and individual level. Trauma is an emotional response to a distressing event. Trauma has an impact on a person's ability to function. To the point that when the event is over, the person continues to experience shock, guilt, shame, and self-blame.

Long term exposure to trauma causes flashbacks, unpredictable emotions and strained relationships. There are three types of traumas. Acute, Complex, and Chronic. Acute trauma stems from a single incident, such as a car accident. Complex trauma comes from multiple traumatic events which are varied by invasive or interpersonal nature. Chronic trauma is caused by violence, domestic or abuse.

Based on research, by the time a child has turned 16 years old, they would have an acute trauma experience. This is important, because when childhood traumas aren't addressed, they carry over into adulthood. With this residue, perhaps problems arise with forming relationships with others or patterns of developing unhealthy relationships become consistent.

Self-Care is valuable to trauma survivors. When practiced, self-care lowers the physiological adrenal surge, which can be lifesaving. According to Andrea Schneider, a licensed clinical social worker she says, "When survivors are able to reprocess and release the traumas, recovery and healing becomes possible." Good self-care strategies can make a huge difference in how well we recover.

At some point in our lives, we will experience being triggered. Often, we are reminded of past traumas causing an overwhelming sense of sadness with anxiety attached to it. Triggers can lead to adverse emotional responses known as emotional triggers. Emotional triggers can come from many different forms, and people are affected in a variety of ways. They are unique to the individual and are based upon many factors. These factors include past experiences, current mental health, substance abuse, and global issues.

We are going to focus on two types of triggers: internal triggers and external triggers. Internal triggers can be memories, physical sensations or emotion. They arise from traumatic events that you have experienced. Also, they come from a deep sense of being lonely, abandoned, or lacking control. It causes emotional pain, and muscle tension. External triggers stem from our environment. They show up in our everyday living experience, and minor inconveniences. These minor inconveniences can be road rage, a neighborhood or community you live in. Researchers believe the brain stores memories from traumatic events, differently from non-traumatic events.

External triggers stem from our environment. They come from your normal everyday life experiences or minor inconveniences. Changes in relationships or ending them. Smells are also associated with external triggers... For example the smell of smoke can trigger a person many years later causing a flashback due to a fire in which that traumatic event occurred. Arguing with a spouse, partner or friend can also bring back memories for someone who has grown up in an abusive household. Self-Care is applicable when triggers are present. When triggered, you can use grounding exercises to connect you to the present moment. Taking in 3 deep breaths or meditating. It's even ok to grab a pillow and scream inside of it.

Have you ever done something and regretted it later? If so, welcome to the regret club. We all have experienced regret. We are all human, having a human experience and regret is normal. It's a natural human emotion. Regret is a very real reaction to a disappointing event in your life. It's a choice you made that can't be changed or something you said you can't take back. It's a feeling that you can't shake as well as a having or intrusive negative emotion that can last for a short or long period of time. Regret prevents a person from re-engaging with life, keeping people isolated and detached and causing people to feel stuck. It impedes your ability to recover quickly from life's events that have become stressful. Regret keeps you bound emotionally for years. Regret shows up in many forms throughout our lives. Such as a loss or missed opportunity. In a nutshell regret is about blaming ourselves for a bad outcome. It's this intense blame that we place on ourselves for our response towards something or someone's negativity.

Regret shows up in such a way that we wish we can undo certain things if given another chance. Research shows, when people have more options over their life's trajectory, regret is experienced. Research also shows that over a short period of time, compared to a long period of time people are likely to regret their actions and mistakes. However, over a long period of time people regret the actions they didn't take. Such as a missed opportunity towards love, not putting family first, and not taking time out for self-care. You may ask why we're talking about regret? Well, the conversation about self-care is overdue. Also, because we are deeply interested in your well-being.

Regret is damaging to your mind, body & soul. It stops a person from bearing fruit or being productive. Your productivity stays very low plus self-blame prevents you from growth. There is a positive side to Regret. As a result, regret can make us do better in the future. It helps us to learn from our experiences and make the necessary changes.

We make decisions constantly, sometimes we must make them quickly, like in a split second. So, when you add the technology component to it. We don't have the time to put enough thought into it. You can love again, you can feel good again, you can start that business again, you can dream again. Why? Because you know yourself a whole lot better through self-care.

There are 4 simple self-care practices that you can do in order to overcome the impact of regret emotionally. First you must practice forgiveness. Forgive yourself and others. The second, practice is to let it go. Allowing yourself the freedom to release it. Third, be intentional about the choices you make. Fourth, write down the lessons you've learned from regrets and rehearse them as needed. Lastly, make sure you're not taking too much of the responsibility or blame for the regret especially when others are involved.

As human beings we are connected by our ability to feel pain. Therefore, this is what brings us here as a collective with time and space. We are present in the very moment right here and right now to heal; our healing process begins simply by letting go. Letting go is self-care. Nobody's life is a straight line of perfection. We all have twists and turns, mountains and valleys. Yet we must let go of all those things that hinder you from growing or becoming a better YOU.

This might be the hardest point for you in this space, for you to do. But lettings go of the trauma, guilt, shame, anger, loss, betrayal, and resentment is essential. Also, you must let go of the self-negativity bias and the shoulda, coulda, woulda's in your life for maximum growth. Practicing letting go is completely up to you. You get to determine if you want to continue to hold on to the hurt and pain or if you want to start your healing journey. Let's do a Letting Go practice together.

1. Offer yourself some compassion and be gentle with yourself.

2. Take 3 deep breaths.

3. Find a comfortable position, place your feet gently on the floor. Eyes closed or open looking down with a soft gaze. Hands placed gently on your lap or to your side, whatever feels comfortable for you, until you feel grounded.

4. Breathe softly, bringing your attention to your breath.

5. Next, recall an image of what you need to let go of. It could be a job, friendship, relationship, unforgiveness, bitterness, a bad habit, or a loss. Whatever it is, feel it. What do you notice? See where it's showing up in your body and hold space for it. Pause for a moment.

6. If something arises for you that's too painful, acknowledge

it, (there is no need for you to hold on to it) bring gentle attention to your breath and breath slowly, Hold it for a moment then let it go.

7. Before you let it go, focus your attention on this moment and say I'm in this moment right here and now. I am prepared to let this go. I want to be healed, I want to be free from pain and suffering. I want to grow, and I

want to be better. Hold it for a few seconds, then let it go!

8. Bring your awareness back to the space, open your eyes, bringing your full attention to your breath.

CHAPTER 6
Taking Care of Your Soul

What is the soul? Do you know what your soul looks like? To define the soul, we'd like to use this simple term. The soul is your mind, emotions, and your will. The soul is your life's center; the core of who you are which is used to express God. However, when we think about self-care and how we can care for ourselves, we must first recognize that we have a soul. Once we understand that, then we must ask the question What is my soul's desire? Due to trauma, inner hurt and deep wounds, our connection to the soul dwindles. Yet deep within our core the soul desires to be healed and to be well.

Your soul is neither passive nor aggressive, it's the link between the physical body and spiritual self. Every experience in life that you've had or will have; and every circumstance from your past up until this point has contributed to the person you are today. A healthy soul will keep you fulfilled and content. As a complete human being it's up to us to

figure out how to heal ourselves.

We have a responsibility to take

care of our soul. Think back for a

moment when you were a child.

Consider the ways in which you were

taught to care for your five-year-old self.

What did that look like? How did you

feel? Were you feeling responsible and

were you rewarded? Did somebody clap

for you and say way to go? As an adult,

soul care isn't always pretty. Often our

five-year-old self shows up wanting to be

nurtured and cared for still. However, there is nobody there clapping and cheering us on. We must look deep within to find the courage to show up for ourselves. This is what self-care is. Having the ability to feed and clothe ourselves in relation to morality we partake in this dynamic experience called reality. We live in a world filled with universal teachers that press upon us the importance of being balanced. Yet our ego gets in the way which causes imbalance overtime.

As we come into the world to share space with others in this vast universe, we arrive with pure intentions. However, as we evolve and grow our interactions with other souls and personalities form conflicts. Each person you meet in life has a soul attached to them. Each soul you meet has had different experiences.

These experiences will look different from your soul's perspective. Our interaction with others teaches us to lead with humility and compassion. This can be done only if we seek out healing for our own souls.

From infancy we are born with an innate ability to trust our parental influencers as well as our familial community. This trust shapes our development as we begin to explore the world around us with curiosity. However, over time, as we encounter multiple personality traits our interpretation of trust gets distorted. This occurs when erroneous situations transpire, time after time thereby making it difficult to move beyond the offense.

A dynamic thing happens, we learn to distrust. Unconsciously, these unpleasant and sometimes painful interactions become deeply rooted in our souls. Painful circumstances and experiences reflect multiple misunderstandings. Mistrust places invisible boundaries within our core; where we become unaware of our limitations deposited by fear. This prevents us from pursuing our dreams, reaching our goals, and from self-improvement. Throughout our lifetime we connect with souls who teach us great lessons about life and trust.

Encountering a distrustful personality is like expecting the unexpected. What we mean by this is as human beings we all tend to be inconsistent. Likewise causing harm to another soul even when we have the purest intentions. Our personalities do conflict with other personalities because the environment in which we were born supports these complexities.

You can change the trajectory of your soul's inner compass by recognizing and reexamining the parts of yourself that need love and compassion. You may have to revisit your inner child, you may have to talk to a therapist, you may have to journal, or sit in silence. Going deep inside the inner core is like diving in the western part of the Pacific Ocean to find that precious pearl. Self-Care for the soul, seeks to heal every broken part, every crack, every tear, and every wound of your soul including trust.

As mentioned earlier, to take care of your soul is to take care of yourself. To take care of yourself is to care for your soul. Soul care is understanding your life's center. At the core of who you are is a healthy soul, and a healthy inner being is necessary without judgment.

<u>Ways to care for your Soul</u>

- Immerse yourself with truth daily. Start by letting the truth in.

- Read inspirational scriptures, affirmations or articles that speak truth to you.

- Speak truth to yourself, no lies.

- Practice gratitude. If practiced daily, this can transform your perspective. Naming your gratitude instantly shifts your soul.

- Be content with what you have, no matter where you are in your life. When you decide to love what you have, right here right now in this moment, something amazing happens in your soul.

- Dream big without limits. Tap into your inner child have a beginner's mind. Dream about all the things you wanted to do without coming up with a reason why you can't. Let your

imagination run wild and free

your soul.

CHAPTER 7
Self-Care and Service to Others

What do you do when self-care practice is not enough? Well, the simplest answer to that question is to serve others. Not just serving them as if you work at a restaurant. The type of service we're talking about is the kind where you get really involved in your community. Organizing outreaches, community engagement activities or even volunteering at your favorite local charity. Passion work is what we're referring to. We're talking about building and maintaining quality relationships that will make a huge impact on your well-being. These connections become a part of a broader community.

Self-Care is community care. There's a famous quote by JKZ which says, "Your interest is best served by recognizing & nurturing the interest of others at the same time." What comes to our mind when reflecting on this quote is a group of individuals who in the 1960's launched more than 35 survival programs. They didn't just launch programs for their community and then walk away. No, they also provided community aid such as education, created health & wellness programs, legal aid, transportation assistance, ambulance services, and distributed free clothes and shoes to the poor living in their community. Doing so was a direct result of self-care practice.

Self-Care is pivotal for managing your psychological, emotional and social well-being. Community care is using the gifts, and resources as well as privilege power to make better the people who are within or without your reach. It could be a colleague, neighbor, a friend, or a member of an organization. Community care also takes shape when practicing anti-racism, ground roots activism, speaking truth to power, donating time, resources and calling out injustices when necessary.

Healthy relationships with others are a cornerstone to happiness and a fulfilled life. Maintaining such relationships can be useful during tough times, also for receiving care and advice. A community is not built overnight, neither are friendships. Having a strong network of support that brings different skills and abilities with them keeps you balanced. Therefore, your support system should provide you with unification from a greater perspective.

What do community support systems look like? To answer that question, we suggest that they are very colorful. For some, support can be in the form of joining new activities, social gatherings, networking events, volunteering, and connecting with those in your community who share common interests. Oftentimes within community interests are the same. Yet many views on how to resolve these complex issues will look different. Keeping an open mind, while being tolerant to differences of opinions allows positivity to shine through.

Mindful listening is about allowing the other person to speak fully authentically without interruptions; not judging what's being said nor having a prepared rebuttal. Support systems thrive off listening to one another. It doesn't matter how difficult the conversation may be, seeing things from someone else's community point of view can help solve so many of the problems that the community is faced with. This is community care at its finest.

Crisis impacts communities in such a way that first responders can't do it alone. When a crisis visits a community, everyone feels it. It shows up in the body. The amygdala part of the brain experiences hijack and from there fight, flight, or freeze responses is activated. Unaware of what to do in those moments, the whole community needs to come together. How else will it wrap its head around what just happened.

Therefore, making sure those who are living in your community feel safe, and protected is self-care. Taking care of each other within the community can help build trust, as well as ongoing community engagement. We can all be leaders in our community by providing the community with resources and ultimately healing. It's up to each person to find their areas of service. Self-care is not an act of selfish intention. Serving others from a filled cup, is a result of your own personal self-care practice. Your community expansion indirectly leans on your inward growth. How you feel, your kindness towards others, and your willingness to give back speaks volumes. For that we say, "Thank you for your service."

CHAPTER 8
Transformative Power of Self-Care

The world around us is changing rapidly. What we see now will no longer be in our tomorrows. You're always transforming, yet it's when you say yes to change that true transformation takes place. Living in the present moment can teach you how to master transformation. How will you transform? Nobody knows for sure. What will your transformation look like? Well, that will depend on how you perceive and practice self-care.

Self-Care practice is a journey. While on this journey of self-care you will begin to experience physical, mental, emotional, and spiritual transformation.

As mentioned in prior chapters, practicing self-care is essential but looks different for each person. However, everyone can become more aware of its impact in their lives. On your journey towards health and wellness, it is vital for you to identify areas in your life where growth is needed.

If you want to transform your life, you will need to change your behaviors by creating new habits. Start by focusing on positive things, appreciating the beauty around you, practicing gratitude, meditating and stimulating your mind. This can assist with achieving your highest-level of self-awareness. How you perceive something to be, and what you're experiencing moving forward must be in total agreement; directly aligned with self. Through transformation, change is inevitable.

Your soul is nudging you to take the path of discovering the real you. Therefore, you will need the courage to apply the self-care practices of finding yourself. Your entire life's trajectory can be transformed simply by practicing self-care.

Much research has been done around the topic of self-care. Some of it may have challenged your belief system or might have triggered some adverse childhood experiences.

Nonetheless by having self-awareness and eradicating self-condemning, self-sabotage, negative self-bias behaviors you've survived overcoming your sufferings.

Inside of us exists a unique interpretation of the world around us. As we experience nature by taking walks, sailing on the ocean, hiking on a hill, sitting by a fire, chasing waterfalls, admiring the colors of rainbows, or simply stopping to smell the roses. We see the beauty in human evolution. The transformational artistry emits energy

allowing one's personal power to shine

brighter than ever.

Again, everyone's self-care

practice will look different. Partly

because our stories are different, also our

childhoods were different. Nevertheless,

each passing day affords you an

opportunity to become more self-aware,

because a new day brings about a fresh

start. Old habits must die, self-doubt

must be abolished, self-judgements

along with guilt and shame must no

longer be the center of your existence. Never speak against yourself. Transformation is your ultimate gift to SELF. Loving you wholeheartedly and authentically is very important as well as being an inspiration to others. There's a saying in society which says, "How you treat You, teaches other people how to treat You." Self-Care is divine. It must always be protected. Eventually as you practice unconditional self-love, you'll become a master of Self-Care. This in turn will spill over to others.

The person you've become, is a direct response of mastering self? Awareness brings you back to truth; total truth, authentic truth more than any mask or identity you've subscribed to. This allows a person to let go of other people's projections, values, or any other idiosyncrasies projected onto them. Self-care helps you wear the opinions of others as a loose garment.

As you transform your journey becomes personal, intentional and purposeful. Respectfully your light shines brighter, illuminating at a higher vibrational frequency.

Our world is shaped by the conditions of man's hearts. If it's full of compassion, empathy, emotional intelligence, kindness, love, pure intentions, generosity, awareness, peace, consideration for others and care; then and only then will we have less resentment, self-inflicted suffering, anger, emotional poisoning, and adverse childhood trauma. Humanity needs a transformative self-care practice. Our society deserves for us to be the best versions of ourselves.

To be the best versions of who we are, we must understand how all that we are, and all that we want to become intersects with what we feel and how we process our emotions. How these emotions show up in our bodies and what we notice. We will do a closing body scan meditation practice. This practice will allow you to focus more throughout your day. It also helps with improving the quality of sleep. Also, for this to be an opportunity to be by yourself and to be with yourself fully. This meditation practice will allow sacred time for nourishment that you well deserve. For a time to send positive energy, attention while connecting to the divine source (God) for strength as well as healing. Letting go of overthinking, critical, judgmental thoughts, accepting what you are feeling in the moment (there is no right way or wrong way to feel). Opening your awareness by watching your body and mind activity.

<u>**Body Scan Meditation**</u>

Find a comfortable position perhaps lying on your back on top of a mat or your bed. (If lying on your back is uncomfortable you may sit down on a chair or stand. Do whatever feels comfortable to feel both relaxed and alert. Allowing your eyes to gently close or looking down with a soft gaze. Gently allow your arms to lay alongside your body. Roll your shoulders back, open your heart space; opening your palms towards the ceiling and allowing your feet to fall away from each other.

Breathing naturally (try not to manipulate it in any way). Bring gentle attention to the breath. Bring your attention to the nostrils or abdomen, notice the in breath, the out breath or that sacred space in between.

Next, bring your attention to the crown of your head, the back of your head & the ears, do you notice any sensations? (Pause)

Next, bring gentle attention to your forehead, the eyes, cheeks, nose, outside your mouth, lips, inside your mouth, the gums, teeth & tongue. (Pause) What do you notice?

Bring your attention to your neck. The back of the neck, the front of the neck, your throat, moving down towards the shoulders, arms, wrist and hands. (Pause) Notice any sensations?

Now, bring your attention to your back, the upper part of the back, the middle of the back, the spine, & the lower back, & glutes. Our back is the part of the body that helps us with bearing the load, to carry the weight and stress in our bodies. Therefore, let's offer extra loving attention to our backs. (Pause) Breathing in on the in breath, breathing out on the out breath.

Now bring gentle attention to the front of your body. To the chest area, the abdomen. Moving down towards the pelvis, the hips, the groin & thighs. (Pause) What's showing up for you?

Now to bring attention to the back of the thighs, the hamstring, moving down to your calves, then back to the front of the legs, bringing attention to the knees, the shins, ankles, all the way down to the top of your feet, bringing attention to the toes, noticing them one by one, bringing attention to the heels of your feet, the bottom & ball of your feet. Our feet are the anchors of the body. They offer us grounding and carry us from place to place, we rely heavily upon them for movement. (Pause)

When you're ready, bring awareness to your entire body whatever state it's in, rest in the stillness and silence of this moment. You are a complete being right here right now. (Pause)

When you are ready, gently bring your full attention back into the open space. Breathing in on the in breath and breathing out on the out breath.

Affirmations

My daily commitment to my self-care

isn't selfish

I choose to let go of negative thoughts

I am strong, empowered and capable of

anything

I am deserving of all the good things in

my life

I am unique and no one can never do it

like me

Every day, I choose to learn more about

my authentic self

I am free of self-doubt and sabotage

I am in control of my negative thoughts

I love, accept and appreciate myself and

my talents

I choose not to take things personally

I must make sure I am regularly taking

care of myself, before I take on too much

to help others.

I am free from expectations and

criticism.

I am making time for self-care

I choose to forgive myself and let go of

my past mistakes.

I am intelligent, courageous and self-confident.

I am patient and gentle with myself and my progress.

I am an independent thinker, not a people pleaser.

I am top priority in my life.

I have every right to say no to anything that makes me feel uncomfortable.

I set healthy boundaries and take extra time to heal if needed.

I honor my intuition and use it as a guide.

I nurture my creative side, as much as

my practical side.

I live with intention and following my

purpose.

I am free from others' negative vibes.

I choose to let go of what I can't control

in my life.

I choose to live in the moment

I am committed to my emotional,

mental, physical and spiritual health.

Self-Care Keys

Get enough sleep

Eat nutritious meals

Exercise

Take technology/social media breaks

Regular medical care

Take vacation/road trip

Make sure to take wellness days off

Be open to intimacy

Book spa days for massages, pedicures & manicures

Take a walk in nature

Journal for self-reflection

Deep breathing, meditation &
mindfulness

Go to therapy

Incorporate aromatherapy for wellness

Join a support group

Think about your positive qualities.

Practice asking for & receiving help

Paint or draw

Attend a symphony or ballet show

Relax in the sun

Gardening

Read a good book

Practice self-compassion & positive self-
talk

Speak words of affirmations

Laugh

Find a hobby

Forgive yourself & others

It's okay to cry

Sing & Dance

Seek spiritual knowledge

Pray

Be playful

Watch the sunrise & sunset

Get to know yourself better

Set goals

Create a vision board

Foster friendships

Manage your finances

Take a break

Volunteer

Spend time with family

Setting boundaries

Learn to say no

Attend professional training

Networking

Go to a cook out

Organize or redecorate a space

Learn to play an instrument

Cuddle with someone you love

INDEX

www.ingramcontent.com/pod-product-compliance
Lightning Source LLC
Chambersburg PA
CBHW021222130726

47988CB00002B/774